K Smith

Slimming with Weights

Ingrid Schultheis

SLIMMING WITH WEIGHTS

A Woman's Guide to Figure Control and Strength Potential

BASED ON THE PROGRAM DESIGNED BY SKIP ARROYO

SAN FRANCISCO BOOK COMPANY, INC.

San Francisco 1977

Library of Congress Cataloging in Publication
Data

Schultheis, Ingrid, 1932–
  Slimming with weights.
  1. Reducing exercises.   2. Weight lifting.
3. Exercise for women.   I. Title.
RA781.6.S38   613.7'1   76-58373
ISBN 0-913374-59-8

Printed in the United States of America
10 9 8 7 6 5 4 3 2 1

Contents

FOREWORD *by Donald G. Watts, M.D.*   7

PREFACE   9

WHY WEIGHTS?   13

EQUIPMENT   21

THE PROGRAM   29

The Beginner's Program   35

The Intermediate Program   63

The Advanced Program   85

APPENDIX OF SPECIAL EXERCISES   107

Acknowledgments   119

Foreword

Like most physicians I have become increasingly alarmed by the number of fad diets, exercise gimmicks, and quick weight-loss methods that have been marketed to the general public over the years. None of them works, many of them are dangerous, and most of them are medically unsound. The result is that those who wish to slim down and keep physically fit only end up with feelings of despair and failure. But when the next crash program appears, they are the first to adopt it, and so the cycle repeats itself again and again.

In talking with my female patients I have come to believe that women are especially vulnerable to this kind of merchandising, because unlike men, they have been conditioned by our society to avoid sports and exercise—particularly the kind of intensive workouts offered by men's gyms. Yet in recent years I think we have begun to see a change in attitude about women and their strength potential, their ability to excel in sports, and their overall stamina and endurance. The idea that women would actually *like* to exercise with weights might have sounded silly a few years ago, but today it's beginning to be taken very seriously indeed. Especially in Berkeley, California, where YMCA Director Skip Arroyo has been helping women work out with weights for the past eight years, it is as if a rediscovery—of health, of fitness, of muscle tone and overall slimness—has been born.

In my practice I have referred many women to Skip Arroyo's gym, and the results have been excellent. The physiological premise of progressive resistance is, first of all, medically sound. Consistent exercising with weights in 45-minute periods—with a day's rest in between—is a very effective and very healthy way to slim the body down. Third, studies have shown that women respond to weight-exercise programs faster than men in terms of increasing strength, but they do *not* develop large muscle mass because of a hormonal (testosterone) difference. Finally, this program is safe: the weights are not heavy enough to cause muscle strain or back injury if used according to instructions.

Slimming with Weights is modeled after Skip Arroyo's ongoing program, and as a practical guide that you can use at home, it is the best I have seen. Given the urgent need in our society for a program of physical fitness that is adaptable to everyday life, and recognizing that for some women the need to lose weight and tone up the body is of utmost importance, I cannot recommend it too highly. You will find that this is the fastest way to slim down possible. I like it because to my knowledge it is the safest and most effective way for busy people to keep physically fit.

Berkeley, California
October 1976

Donald G. Watts, M.D.

Preface

Although this book is for all women who want to slim down fast, I would like to address a few words here to women like myself who are moving into middle age and seem to have no time in their busy schedules to pay attention to how much exercise they're getting or where their energy is going. If you are fatigued much of the time, or if you have tried swimming, tennis, jogging, or other sports to "keep fit" and ended up frustrated or drained of energy, please read on.

This book is the result of my own search for an exercise program that would really work. As a working mother with no time to "exercise for the sake of exercise," I needed an efficient program that not only would keep my figure trim and my energy level high, but would make me *feel* well—healthy and active and ready to enjoy life anew. I wanted a program that would give me a good, solid workout with quick, positive results—all in a minimal period of time.

Nevertheless, when I first heard of a new weight-exercise program for women that was reputed to work wonders, even for middle-aged and elderly women, I was reluctant to look into it. The thought of lifting weights was associated in my mind with bulging, oversized muscles and thick necks, a "Mr. Universe" image that was better suited to male weight lifters than to busy women. Then one day I went to the YMCA in Berkeley, California, and it was there that I first encountered this program of weight exercises for women.

Astonished, I saw dozens of supple, slim, feminine, wonderfully healthy women of all ages working with weights of all shapes and sizes. None of them had bulging muscles or overdeveloped limbs or bore any resemblance to the stereotype of male weight lifters, even though several had really "gotten into" weight lifting and had moved on to other programs where they were able to "press" as much as 80–90 pounds. The youngest woman there was 16 and the oldest was 81. The weights were not big, bulky barbells at all, but small and compact hand weights, boots, and bars. Women with back problems had been placed on a special program that now enabled them to lift, bend, stretch, and exercise with weights in ways they had never thought possible before. And women with bursitis and arthritis (who told me they could not even lift their arms to shoulder level before starting the program) were now moving weights in giant circles over their heads.

I tried it, and the effect was instantaneous. I discovered dormant muscles; I could actually feel my arm and leg muscles tensing, working, firming. My muscles lifted without strain and moved with vibrancy and renewed strength. It was invigorating rather than exhausting, replenishing rather than draining, and after 45 minutes I walked out of that gym with a bounce to my step I hadn't felt in years.

At times, I suppose, the sessions that followed must have sounded like self-congratulatory testimonials—and slightly evangelical ("I've gotten rid of the

10

flab around my middle" . . . "My friends can't believe my new figure" . . . "Look at this! I've lost an inch a month—I'm a whole new me!").

That was three years ago. Since then I have been exercising regularly for only 45 minutes every other day, sometimes less, with little other exercise in between. Today I am physically healthier, more agile, and stronger than most women in their twenties. I am rarely fatigued and almost constantly energized—and "miraculously" I have not fallen prey to middle-age spread. Every woman who has participated in the program feels the same way, including those who are elderly or afflicted with back problems or bursitis—and so will you.

Try it. Throw out those "quickie/crash" books and gimmicks and feel your muscles *work* for a change. Commit yourself to less than three hours a week and stick to it. It's not just that the inches will seem to melt away. There is also that marvelous discovery that your body can be as fit, as strong, as healthy, and as slim as it ever was or as you ever wanted it to be.

Good health and slim, agile bodies are not a "gift of youth" but a result of constant personal care. If you've tried other methods and failed because too much time and exertion resulted in too few rewards, try this program. There is no faster way, no easier way, no more rewarding way to slim down, shape up, and feel better than this simple program of exercising with weights.

Why Weights?

Though traditionally "for men only," exercising with weights is an extremely effective way for women to lose inches and shape firm, feminine figures. Imagine trimming, slimming, and losing weight faster than you ever have before; toning and firming a shapelier figure than you ever thought possible; discovering untapped resources of strength that allow you to move heavy equipment without having to wait for help—and all of this possible through a simple, efficient, and exciting new program that requires less than *three hours a week*.

This is the program that has been tested and perfected over the past eight years at the Berkeley, California YMCA, where director Skip Arroyo works with women from 16 to 81 on a weight-exercise program of her own design. She knows how women can take inches off their waists, thighs, and legs in the fastest, easiest, most efficient way possible; how women who think of themselves as weak or frail or stiff can develop strength and agility they never knew they had. Tennis players, swimmers, and joggers find that working with weights increases stamina and endurance as well as enjoyment and competence in all physical activities. Most of all, women who have tried and failed at

13

other methods—from "cellulite" exercises to air force calisthenics, from crash diets to clotheslines-on-pulleys or expensive machines—find that *this* is the program that works. *This* is the program that women never have to talk themselves into doing: they continue with enthusiasm and vigor even after they've lost the inches they wanted to lose and discovered the resources of strength they never knew they had—and so can you.

You need nothing more than the materials you already have at home and the willingness to "work out" for 45 minutes *every other* day. But first let's examine some of the questions many women ask when they first consider exercising with weights.

Q: Why is exercising with weights more effective than other exercise programs?
A: The principle behind this program is called *progressive resistance.* This means that the added resistance provided by the weights causes your muscles to put forth a greater amount of energy than they would in a conventional program of calisthenics. You can test this right now by raising your hand to your shoulder, an effortless gesture that is the result of flexing the bicep. Now put a heavy book in your hand and raise it to your shoulder again. Feel the difference? Your muscles must work harder to overcome the resistance of the added weight. Thus the key to this program is to *maximize* muscular effort within a *minimum* period of time. The process works so fast that you will very quickly be able to lift the weight more times than you did at first, and soon you will be able to lift it almost without effort: this is because your strength has built up to the point that you must increase the resistance by adding more weight in

order to maximize muscular effort again. The progression from light to heavy weights and few to many repetitions not only speeds up the toning and slimming process, it also results in a substantial increase in strength and endurance.

Each exercise in this program works on specific muscles, so if you have problem areas which you especially want to slim and strengthen, you can select the appropriate exercises and concentrate on them. Accordingly, each exercise is introduced with a brief description explaining which muscles or parts of the body it is designed to benefit.

Q: Will I develop bulky, brawny muscles?

A: No. Experience has shown—and scientific experiments have proven—that most women who exercise with weights simply do *not* develop bulky muscles. It is the predominantly male hormone, testosterone, which is responsible for the development of bulky muscles in men. Testosterone is also present in women, but usually in amounts too low to increase muscle size substantially. If you're skeptical, take a look at the photographs in this book of our model Jody, who began working with weights about four years ago. After a year, seeking a greater challenge, she started on a more strenuous weightlifting program and now works out regularly with weights as heavy as 60 to 90 lbs. Jody reports that working with heavier weights "gives me a great sense of physical *and* mental well-being without worrying about becoming muscle-bound."

Q: Will these exercises give me a masculine appearance?

A: No. As Dr. Lawrence Morehouse, Director of the Human Performance Laboratory at the University of California at Los Angeles (and author of *Total Fitness*) has said, "The common idea that weightlifting will make a woman mannish-looking is groundless." In fact, Dr. Morehouse states, "A woman can be made more womanly by this exercise, which was formerly considered to be exclusively masculine. Her clothes will fit her better, and she will feel like holding her head up and shoulders back." Working with weights, Dr. Morehouse concludes, can "flatten and firm up flabby stomachs, improve muscle tone and carriage, and strengthen the heavy muscles under the breasts and thus improve the bustline."

Q: Will I injure myself working with weights?
A: In this program you will *never* use any weights sufficiently heavy to cause bodily injury. If a particular exercise is difficult for you, or if you find that increasing the size of the weight causes strain or pain, then you should STOP. Go back to the lighter weight for the present and make the heavier weight your new goal. Some women prefer to alternate exercises for the upper part of the body with exercises for the legs and lower body. Such an approach allows one area to rest from intense muscular exertion while another area gets a real work out.

   If you have doubts about your strength potential (and many women do) and fear that you are too weak to participate in weight-resistive exercises, then this program is *especially* for you. Rapidly and dramatically it will increase your ability to carry heavy packages, move furniture, and work with heavy equipment.

Q: But I have a weak back!

A: Then it is doubly important for you to exercise with weights and to strengthen those vulnerable muscles and joints that are giving you trouble now. Of course, everyone should check with a doctor about any new exercise program to make sure you're in good health. If you are already under a doctor's care, you should ask your physician specifically about working with weights. If your problem is back strain, back aches, or weak back muscles, begin with the special exercises on page 109 and progress to the exercises you can perform without strain. (See "A Word of Encouragement," p. 33.)

Q: Will these exercises make my muscles sore and stiff?

A: You may notice some muscle soreness on the day after you have begun, especially in those muscles that are weak from years of disuse. But a certain amount of soreness can be interpreted as a good sign—it tells you that you have begun to revitalize weakened and long-neglected muscles. If you do experience soreness on the day following your first day of exercising with weights, then you should also exercise on this day and on the following day as well. By exercising with weights for three consecutive days you will work out the initial soreness and will be ready to proceed to the every-other-day program.

As for normal stiffness, the warm-up exercises at the beginning of each section are specifically designed to limber up your muscles and to work the stiffness out of your body. Most of us, whether we know it or not, are simply riddled with tension and need to work into using the weights for maximum effect with minimum strain.

Q: Will exercising with weights make me tired?

A: Emphatically NO. These exercises not only increase your muscular strength, they also increase your endurance as well. In fact, using weights with these exercises enables you to release excess energy so that you can relax and sleep better. And since tension is often the reason you feel fatigued or tired, after exercising you will feel more exuberant, less tired, and more ready to enjoy life.

Q: What about "dimpled" fat on the thighs and upper arms, or loose, hanging flab, or "puckered" loose skin?

A: It is a *myth* that once women reach a certain age they cannot rid themselves of "dimpled" or "puckered" fat. What *is* true is that working with weights benefits your entire body, resulting in "better muscle tone, therefore less flab," as Dr. Dorothy Harris, exercise physiologist at Pennsylvania State University, explains. As muscles tighten and inches are lost, the dimples and puckers will gradually disappear.

Q: Does this program require a special diet?

A: If losing weight is your goal, you should certainly avoid foods that are high in calories, starches, sugars, and fats, but basically this is a common sense approach that requires no "crash diets" or special regimens. Working with weights, combined with a sensible diet, will result in losing inches where you

18

need to lose them and gaining strength and endurance in long-neglected muscles. You can speed up this process by eating more protein and less starch than you usually do. It's as simple as that.

Q: How much weight or inches can I lose and at what rate?

A: In this program you can expect to lose an inch a month wherever you need to lose it if you commit yourself to doing these exercises for 45 minutes every other day and watch (but not necessarily change) your diet. For women who conscientiously cut back on their calorie intake, working with weights can help them lose pounds faster than other approved programs. But remember *this* program is designed to help you lose inches; the emphasis is on slimming rather than on losing pounds—which for many women is the same thing. If losing weight is your goal, combine this program with the special diet your doctor has developed for you. Then not only will you feel better as you lose weight, you will also look better, slimmer, and trimmer much faster than you ever thought possible.

Q: But I hate to exercise!

A: So do most people until they begin working with weights, as you'll see. It is because most exercise programs require too much "flapping around" with too few rewards that most of us get discouraged very soon and give up. Remember that the weights cause your muscles to work harder with each movement, so you won't have to make as many movements to achieve results. If you have failed to sustain interest in other exercise programs, it's probably not your fault. No one can be expected to remain committed to a boring and lengthy daily procedure that makes you wait too long for too few results. When you work with weights your whole attitude about exercise will change because you'll see the results quickly and you'll feel your muscles toning up with each movement. Further, this is not a daily but an *every-other-day* routine that gives your body time to rest and relax between sessions. You'll probably find yourself looking forward to each 45-minute period because of its positive effect on both your mental and physical well-being and its long-range results in slimming down and toning up *every* part of your body.

Equipment

Without realizing it, you may already have all the equipment you need to start working with weights right in your own home. So before you decide to purchase a set of weights or make your own at home, walk through your house with an eye to finding compact, weighty objects that are easily grasped and manipulated. Heavy hiking boots or ski boots weigh anywhere from 2 to 5 pounds and are perfect for use as hand weights and weight boots in the Beginner's Program. Steam irons or other small utensils will also serve as hand weights for beginners, as will heavy books if your grip is strong enough.

TO CONSTRUCT YOUR OWN WEIGHTS:

When you reach the Advanced Program, you will need to use weights that are specifically designed for this program. For the Beginner's and Intermediate Program, however, it is easy—and inexpensive—to construct your own weights, as again you probably already have many of the necessary items:

a broomstick
some fine-grained sand

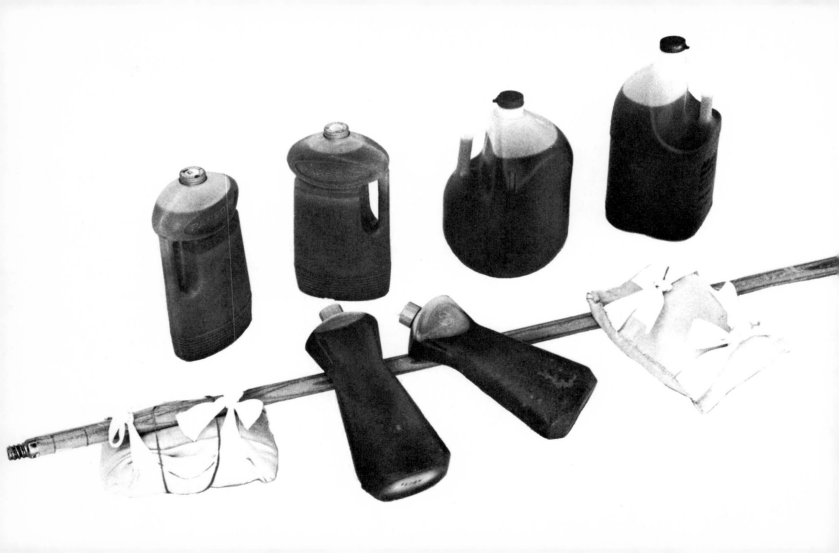

several empty plastic bottles (with handles for easy gripping—try empty bottles of laundry bleach, detergent, distilled water, etc.)
4 pieces of 12 x 12 inch sturdy fabric such as denim (an easy way is to use the pantlegs from an old pair of jeans)
8 12-inch strips of strong ribbon
sturdy rubber bands

To make a 3-lb. weight:

Fill a 48 fluid oz. plastic bottle with water. Screw the top on tightly.

To make a 5-lb. weight:

Put 6½ cups of sand into a 56 fluid oz. plastic bottle.

To make a 10-lb. weight:

Fill a 1 gal. plastic bottle with sand, leaving a 1″ air space at the top.

To make weight shoes:
(You can also use these bags as hand weights by slipping your hands through the ribbon, palm side next to the cloth.)

Make a bag from a 12 x 12 inch piece of sturdy cloth. Make the seams strong and be sure to leave one side open. Fill a double plastic bag with 4 cups of sand and close it tightly with wire ties or rubber bands. Put this sand-filled plastic bag into the cloth bag and sew the cloth bag tightly closed. At each corner of the bag, sew on a strong ribbon 12 inches

23

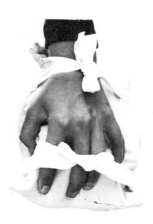

long. You now have a 3-lb. weight to tie on top of your shoe. To make a 5-lb. weight shoe, follow the instructions for a 3-lb. weight shoe above, except fill the double plastic bag with 6½ cups of sand.

To make an exercise bar:

Take a broom stick and tie a 5-lb. bag at each end. Use some rubber bands around the bags to make sure that they are attached securely.

For a bench:

A garden type will do fine, or you can use a few stools placed close together.

TO PURCHASE YOUR WEIGHTS:

Purchasing the equipment needed for this program is quite simple and, in the long run, quite inexpensive. Although the weight sets you'll find in most large department stores, well-equipped sporting goods stores, or gym supply stores can be very costly, you can easily combine many of the units of a smaller set and cut costs considerably.

It is best to avoid ready-made plastic-covered dumbbells of the 3-lb. or 5-lb. size because you cannot add or remove weights from these units. Instead,

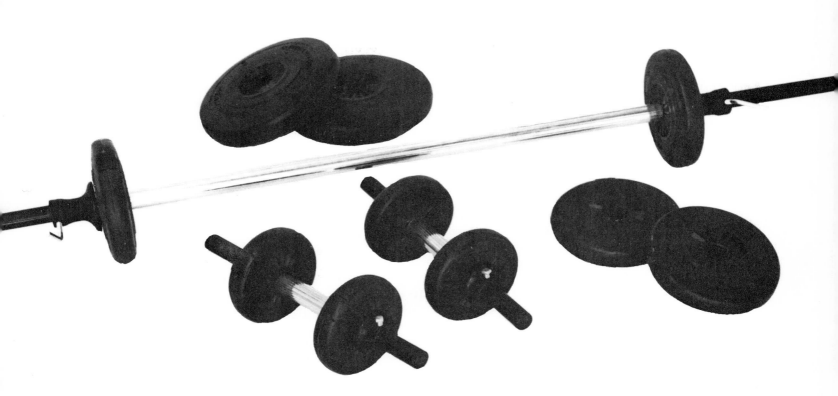

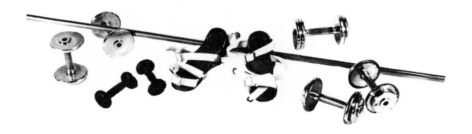

look for a set of weights that includes 1 long bar (about 60 inches) and 2 short bars (about 15 inches) with adjustable pairs of discs weighing 2½ lb., 5 lb., and 10 lb. Do not worry if the weights which you buy are ½ lb. or 1 lb. lighter than the exercises in this book call for. Anything reasonably close to the stipulated weight size will be both acceptable and effective. A 2½- or 5-lb. disc can be held separately in the hand to serve as a dumbbell (arthritics can use heavy rubber strips to secure the discs to each hand). You can also make these discs double as weight shoes by inserting a heavy rubber strip through the hole in the middle of the disc and strapping it onto your foot. Thus if you prefer not to buy weight boots (which cost about $15), you can simply purchase a small weight set of bars and discs. Such a set usually costs $25 to $30 and will be adequate for the entire program.

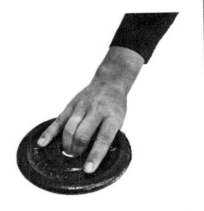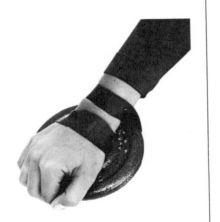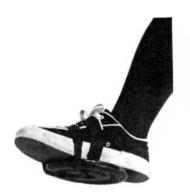

27

The Program

There are three stages to the program—Beginner's, Intermediate, and Advanced. Each stage is designed to make you progressively stronger, but *all* stages will help you lose unwanted inches and build up neglected, sagging muscles. Remember that the principle behind this program is "progressive resistance" (see p. 14). The longer you work with increasingly heavy weights, the stronger you will become and the faster your muscles will tone up and slim you down. So do not try to rush through the first stages with the idea of speeding up the effects of the overall program, because the results you want will begin with the first stage: you will feel stronger, healthier, more agile and alive. You will discover muscles you never thought you had, and you will notice a definite slimming-down—a new litheness to your body. Your clothes will fit better and your posture will improve, and you will be astonished to find that those heavy packages, items of furniture, children, or equipment will suddenly seem lighter and easier to pick up and carry. All of this will be noticeable to you within the first few weeks.

By the end of a full month you will notice a *measurable* loss, in inches, of unwanted fat. So take a moment on the first day to measure yourself and record your statistics on the chart on page 30.

DATE STARTED: _____

Measurements	At the Beginning	After 1 Month	After 2 Months	After 3 Months	After 4 Months	After 5 Months	After 6 Months	After 7 Months	After 8 Months	After 9 Months	After 10 Months
BUST											
WAIST											
ABDOMEN											
HIPS											
THIGHS											
CALF											
UPPER ARM											
WEIGHT											

30

Note the date you start the program and be certain *not* to measure or weigh yourself again until a full month has passed. On that day you can actually start thinking about buying clothes in a size smaller than you're wearing now. Each month's measurements should provide you with renewed incentive to continue working with weights into the next month, but even after you have lost the inches you needed to lose, you'll want to keep going. The overall feeling of total health, renewed vitality, and streamlined fitness won't let you stop.

A WORD ABOUT BREATHING

Anyone can lift a few weights up and down once or twice. But when you get to the eighth or ninth time, or when in the Intermediate or Advanced Program you are working hard to reach the fifteenth or twentieth time, you'll want to give those muscles all the help you possibly can. One way is to keep your blood circulating throughout your body in order to reach those muscles that are doing the heaviest work. By breathing deeply and rhythmically, you can actually provide the heart with a "secondary pump." This is necessary because holding your breath in the midst of exertion slows the flow of blood. So make a point to breathe deeply each time you move those weights, and to follow specific breathing instructions where indicated. You'll soon discover how invaluable rhythmic breathing can be to maintaining your endurance, increasing your strength, and slimming your body down to the exact proportions you want.

31

A WORD ABOUT STRAIN

Do not worry if the weights seem heavier and more difficult to move as you complete each exercise—in fact, that's the point. If it takes an all-out effort to lift the weights one last time, or if you find yourself sweating because of the effort needed to keep your muscles working as they move the weights, all the better. Remind yourself that it will only last a few minutes more and that the more you exert yourself in this concentrated effort, the faster your body will tone up and slim down. What you are feeling is not strain (injury by overuse or overexertion) but good old-fashioned hard work, a lost value in our sedentary lifestyles today and one that will pay off in benefits you can measure—by the inch!

Remember too, however, that there is no benefit to working in pain. If it hurts, you should STOP and go back to lighter weights until you build up your strength to continue the program.

A WORD ABOUT TENSION AND RELAXATION

Because exercising with weights requires your muscles to work hard and to use up much more energy than other calisthenic programs, it also relaxes more effectively. Tension is the result of a continuous, low-level contraction of muscles that are constantly prepared for action but are never allowed to act. Exercising with weights not only releases tension throughout the entire body, it is especially helpful for working out tension in the shoulder and neck areas, where many office workers are particularly prone to develop tension pain such as stiff necks, sore shoulders, and back aches. Such tension-generated aches and pains can be easily prevented by exercising with weights on a regular basis.

A WORD OF ENCOURAGEMENT TO SUFFERERS OF BACK ACHES AND BACK PROBLEMS

If you are under a doctor's care because of a specific ailment in your back, you must of course check with your physician before beginning any new exercise program. But for those many millions of women who go through each day with minor back aches and pains, exercising with weights is a godsend: it strengthens the attendant muscles of the spine, improves posture, alleviates aches and tension in the lower back, and helps to prevent what many doctors believe is the worst danger for backs—the slipped disc. If you are in this category, note the special exercises in the Appendix and do these first. Then proceed through the program and omit those exercises that women with back problems should *not* do.

Before you start the Beginner's Program, take a moment to think about how you usually pick up your children, or lift heavy pieces of furniture or equipment. Do you bend from the waist and pull (wrong!), or do you bend from the knees and *lift* (right!)? As you develop new resources of strength in this program, you'll find it easier to lift the 10-lb. and 20-lb. bar, but don't stop there. Make this new strength work for you everywhere you can—you'll be amazed at the weight you can lift without back strain and the new way your body will "stand tall."

All set? Let's begin.

The Beginner's Program

Choose a quiet place where you will not be disturbed. You should have sufficient space around you to be able to extend your arms and legs fully in all directions. Wear a pair of leotards or loose clothes that permit you to stretch and move freely.

The program is designed to work on all muscles of the body, starting from the top and working down. If you wish to concentrate on specific problem areas, do all of the exercises in the program first, then go back and perform those exercises that are particularly helpful to you. Remember the principle of progressive resistance: keep trying to increase the number of times you perform each exercise so that you can more quickly firm and slim your body as you go along.

The full program will take 45 minutes to complete, but as you become more familiar with the structure and requirements of these exercises, you may be able to move through the program more quickly. (If you're short of time, do not skip any of the exercises; instead, cut down on the number of repetitions in each.) Remember that if you feel soreness in your muscles following the first day of exercise, then exercise again on this day, and on the following day as well. By exercising for three consecutive days, you should be able to work out most of the stiffness. You will then be ready to begin exercising on an every-other-day basis, allowing your muscles a day of rest between sessions.

You may find that your body is not ready to do the boot exercises immediately when you begin this program. If so, give yourself about two weeks to get your legs into shape by doing only Exercises 1–16. Then for the next two weeks, skip Exercise 16 and add the boot exercises to the full routine.

The Beginner's Program lasts four weeks. If you feel strong enough to proceed to the Intermediate Program earlier, by all means do so, making certain that none of the exercises in that program cause you any pain or soreness.

Once you are familiar with the sequence of the exercises, use this checklist for quick reference:

Warm-Ups
1. Bending: repeat 5 to 10 times.
2. Dumbbell Swings: 1 5-lb. weight, repeat 5 to 10 times.
3. Dumbbell Bends: 2 5-lb. weights, repeat 10 to 15 times each side .

Upper Body
4. Dumbbell Bench Press: 2 5-lb. weights, repeat 8 to 15 times.
5. Bent Arm Lateral: 2 5-lb. weights, repeat 8 to 15 times.
6. Overhead to Hips: 2 3-lb. weights, repeat 8 to 15 times.

Arms	7. Curls: 2 5-lb. weights, repeat 10 to 15 times.
	8. Lean Over Push–Back: 2 3-lb. weights, repeat 10 to 15 times.
	9. Dips From Bench: repeat up to 10 times.
Waist and Stomach	10. Bar Twist: 10-lb. bar, repeat 10 to 15 times.
	11. Bar Twist Seated: 10-lb. bar, repeat 10 to 15 times.
	12. Twisting Sit-Ups: repeat 10 to 15 times.
	13. Bent Leg Raises: repeat 10 to 15 times.
Hips, Thighs, and Legs	14. Leg Lunges: 2 5-lb. weights, repeat 5 times.
	15. Calf Raises: repeat 10 times.
	16. Leg Lifts: repeat 10 times each leg.
	17. Leg Extension Back: 3-lb. boots, repeat 8 to 12 times each leg.
	18. Leg Raises on Side: 3-lb. boots, repeat 8 to 12 times each leg.
	19. Leg Lifts from Bench: 3-lb boots, repeat 8 to 12 times each leg.
	20. Leg Circles: 3-lb. boots, repeat 8 to 12 times each leg.
	21. Leg Lifts with Boots: 3-lb boots, repeat 5 to 10 times each leg.

1 • Bending

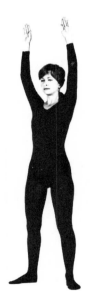

This is a good exercise for limbering the legs and spine.

Stand with your feet shoulder-width apart and your arms stretched above your head.

Stretch upward as far as you can—imagine that you are trying to touch the ceiling.

Then bend at the waist and touch the floor with your hands while keeping your legs straight.

Bounce 3 times in this position and then straighten up.

Repeat 5 to 10 times.

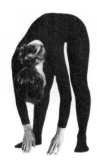

Don't worry if you're a little stiff and cannot easily reach the floor with your hands. Just bend down as far as is comfortable. Be patient. You will reach the floor in good time.

2 • Dumbbell Swings *

In addition to limbering and relaxing, this exercise helps to slim the hips and waist.

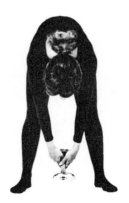

Hold a 5-lb. weight with both hands and stand with your feet shoulder-width apart. (To avoid straining the back, never use more than a 5-lb. weight for this exercise.)

Keeping your legs straight, bend down at the waist.

Make a circle with your arms—sideways, overhead, and then down.

Reverse and make another complete circle.

Repeat 5 times. Gradually increase to 10.

* If you have back problems, replace this exercise with the special back exercises on pages 109-112.

40

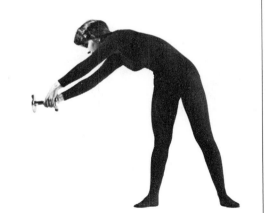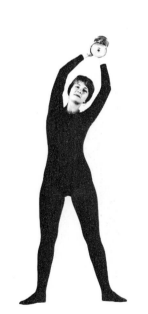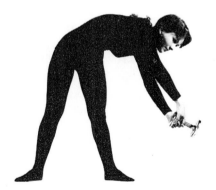

41

3 • Dumbbell Bends

This exercise stretches and slims the waist and hips.

Holding a 5-lb. weight in each hand, stand with your legs apart.

Bend from side to side, keeping your back straight. Let the weight pull you down to the side *as far as possible*. You will be able to feel your side muscles stretch.

Repeat 10 times to each side. Gradually increase to 15.

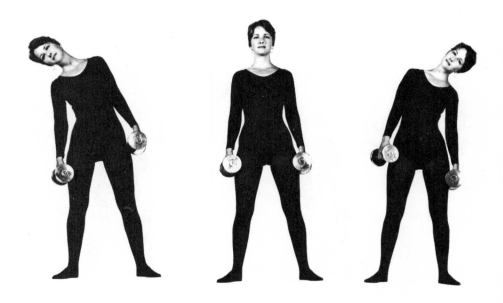

4 • Dumbbell Bench Press

This exercise firms your bustline, slims your upper arms, and gives you shapelier shoulders.

With a 5-lb. weight in each hand, lie on your back on a bench.

Start with your arms straight up. Inhale deeply as you bring the weights down alongside your bustline.

Now exhale as you return arms to starting position.

Repeat 8 times. Gradually increase to 15.

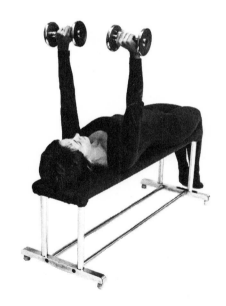

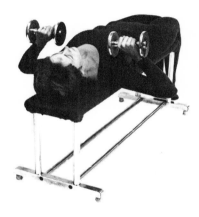

Take your time and don't hurry. Feel your lungs expand and your shoulders loosen up.

43

5 • Bent Arm Lateral

Exhale as you slowly return arms to starting position.

Repeat 8 times. Gradually increase to 15.

This exercise is excellent for toning arm muscles, firming the bustline, and increasing strength.

With a 5-lb. weight in each hand, lie on your back on a bench.

Start with your arms straight up, weights facing each other. Inhale deeply as you lower arms to the sides with elbows slightly bent. To avoid straining, do not drop arms below bench level.

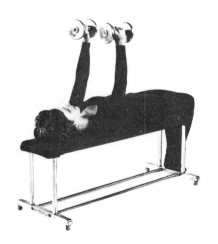

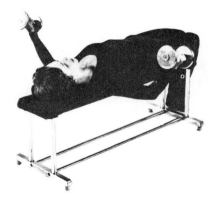

44

6 • Overhead to Hips *

This exercise firms the bustline and the shoulder area.

With a 3-lb. weight in each hand, lie on your back on a bench.

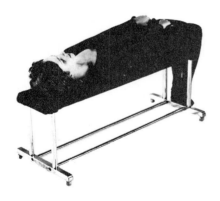

Start with your arms straight down, weights resting on your thighs.

Keeping your arms straight, inhale deeply as you raise them up over your body and then over your head.

Now exhale completely as you trace a circle in the air by moving your arms out and away from your body and then back down to the starting position.

Repeat 8 times. Gradually increase to 15.

* If you have arthritis or bursitis in the shoulder area, do not make the circle. Instead, raise your arms up over your body only, and then return to starting position.

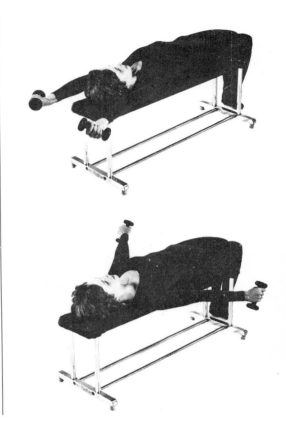

45

7 • Curls

This simple but very effective exercise firms and strengthens the front arm muscles.

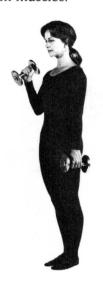

Stand holding a 5-lb. weight in each hand.

Raise the dumbbell in your right hand to the level of your right shoulder.

Now lower the right hand weight to starting position while you bring the weight in the left hand up to the level of the left shoulder. Return left hand and weight to original position.

Because this exercise is so easy to do, you may be tempted to do it quickly. You will achieve maximum benefits, however, only if you perform this exercise at a moderate speed.

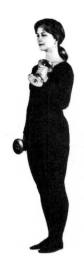

Repeat 10 times. Gradually increase to 15.

8 • Lean over Push-Back

This exercise shapes and strengthens the backs of the upper arms and the upper back muscles. It is also wonderful for flabby underarms.

Stand with a 3-lb. weight in each hand.

Holding arms close to your body, bend forward at the waist until your back is parallel to the floor. Lift your elbows as high as possible.

Keeping elbows in this position, swing your forearms back and up behind your torso. Feel those neglected muscles at the back of your upper arms come to life when you do this exercise.

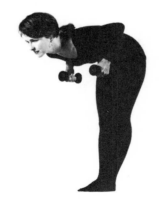

Return to starting position.

Repeat 10 times. Gradually increase to 15.

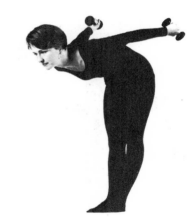

47

9 • Dips from Bench

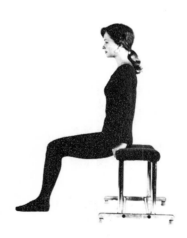

This exercise firms the upper arms and upper back, improves posture, and strengthens the entire upper body.

Sit on a bench or chair and grasp the edge with your hands. Your feet should be on the floor and your knees should be bent.

Supporting yourself with your arms, raise your body to the full length of your arms.

Then lower yourself until your buttocks almost touch the floor.

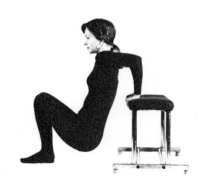

Return to starting position.

Repeat 10 times.

10 • Bar Twist

This exercise slims the upper waist, helps to flatten the tummy, and improves posture.

Rest a 10-lb. bar across your shoulders behind your head.

With a wide grip on the bar and a wide stance, twist your torso rhythmically from side to side.

To maximize the slimming effect on the waist, your face and hips should remain stationary, facing forward at all times. You'll feel your stomach muscles stretch and breathe as if for the first time!

Repeat 10 times. Gradually increase to 15.

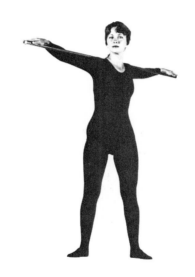

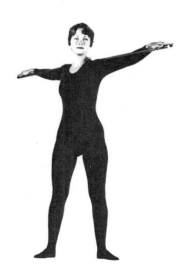

49

11 • Bar Twist Seated

This exercise slims and firms the lower waist.

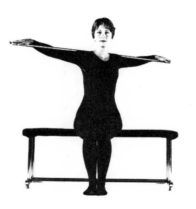

Sit on a bench and rest a 10-lb. bar across your shoulders behind your head.

With a wide grip on the bar, twist your torso rhythmically from side to side. Keep hips as stationary as possible.

Repeat 10 times. Gradually increase to 15.

12 • Twisting Sit-Ups

This exercise strengthens the abdominal muscles and flattens the stomach.

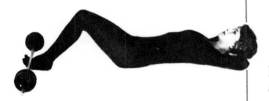

Lie on the floor and hook your feet under a weight or a piece of heavy furniture. Your knees should be bent—this forces the stomach muscles to work hard and eliminates back strain.

Clasp your hands behind your head and sit up.

Now twist your torso and bend forward so that you can touch your left elbow to your right knee.

Twist to the other side to touch right elbow to the left knee.

Return to starting position slowly.

Repeat 10 times. Gradually increase to 15.

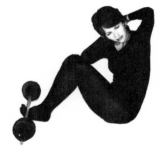

If this exercise seems strenuous at first, instead of clasping your hands behind your head, try raising your arms over your head while you sit up.

51

13 • Bent Leg Raises *

This exercise strengthens the abdominal muscles and is great for flattening the stomach.

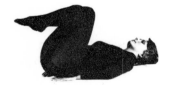

Lie on your back on the floor.

Draw your knees to your chest. Then straighten your legs toward the ceiling.

With legs straight, bring them slowly back down to the floor.

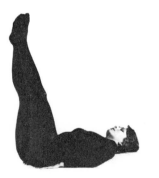

Repeat 10 times. Gradually increase to 15.

* If you have back problems, replace this exercise with the special back exercises on pages 109-112.

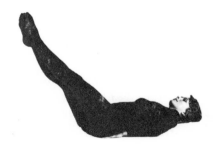

52

14 • Leg Lunges *

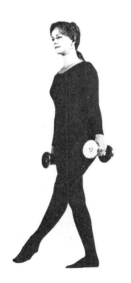

This exercise improves posture and develops youthful suppleness in all the lower body muscles from the hip to the foot.

Stand holding a 5-lb. weight in each hand.

From standing position lunge forward with one leg, bending both knees.

Bend rear knee as far as possible, but do not touch the floor.

Hold this position for several seconds and notice the pull in the back of the leg and at the front of the thigh.

Step back to starting position. Then lunge forward with the other leg.

Return to starting position.

Repeat 5 times.

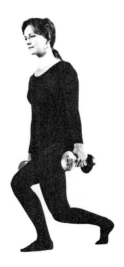

* If you have knee problems, replace this exercise with the special knee exercise on p. 113.

15 • Calf Raises

This exercise, which will seem almost childishly effortless, is marvelous for strengthening calf muscles and improving posture.

Stand with the balls of your feet on a thin board or book (about 1½ inches thick). Your heels should be touching the floor.

Raise your heels while keeping the front of your feet stationary on the board.

Lower your heels to the floor.

Repeat 10 times.

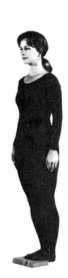

16 • Leg Lifts

If you feel ready to use boots, skip this exercise and proceed.

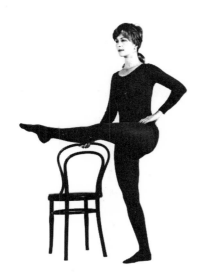

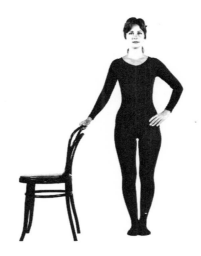

This exercise releases tension in the legs, thighs, and buttocks. It also shapes and strengthens the thighs and buttocks.

Stand holding on to the back of a chair with one hand. Place your weight on the leg which is next to the chair and lift the other leg forward. Keep both legs straight as you do this. Lower your leg to the floor. Then lift it out to the side.

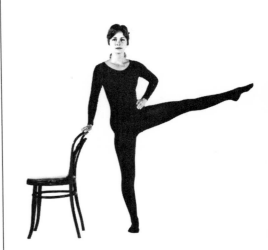

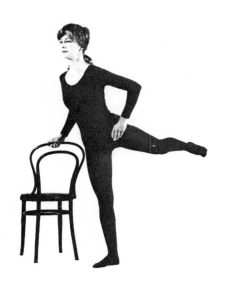

To maximize the slimming effect of this exercise, use a kicking motion to raise your leg as high as possible on each lift.

Repeat 10 times with each leg.

Lower your leg again. Then lift it back behind you. Return to your starting position.

17 • Leg Extension Back *

This exercise slims hips and thighs, strengthens abdominal muscles, and firms the neck.

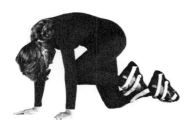

With 3-lb. boots on, begin by kneeling with hands flat on the floor, arms straight, chin tucked down.

Bring your right knee forward and try to touch your chin with it.

Then stretch your right leg back and up as much as you can, raising your chin at the same time.

Return to your starting position.

Don't hurry as you do this exercise. Allow your muscles to stretch slowly.

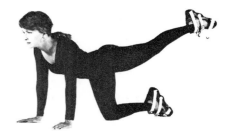

Repeat 8 times with each leg. Gradually increase to 12.

* If you have back problems, replace this exercise with the special back exercises on pages 109-112.

57

18 • Leg Raises on Side

This exercise slims and firms thighs, legs, and buttocks.

With 3-lb. boots on, lie on your side on the floor and rest your head on your hand.

58

Raise your leg up as high as possible and then lower it slowly to starting position.

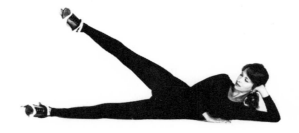

You may find it increasingly difficult to raise each leg as you approach the eighth lift, but keep trying; this exercise and the ones that follow really take those inches off!

Repeat 8 times with each leg. Gradually increase to 12.

19 • Leg Lifts from Bench

This exercise shapes and firms the buttocks.

With 3-lb. boots on, kneel your right leg on a bench as shown, making sure that your foot is over the end for good support. Your left foot should be resting on the floor.

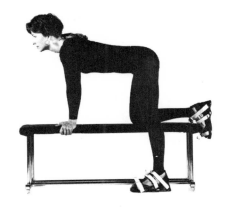

Keeping your left leg straight, lift it until it is parallel with the bench.

Return to starting position.

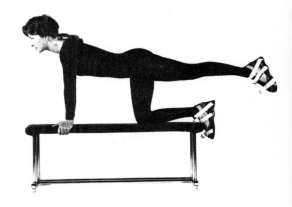

Repeat 8 times with each leg. Gradually increase to 12.

59

20 • Leg Circles

Do this exercise in a nice, easy rhythm. Feel the tightness disappear as the hip joint loosens up and moves easily.

This exercise slims and shapes the hips.

With 3-lb. boots on, stand holding on to the back of a chair with your right hand.

Make a large circle in the air with your left leg, keeping it straight.

When you have completed the circle, rest your foot on the floor.

Repeat 8 times with each leg. Gradually increase to 12.

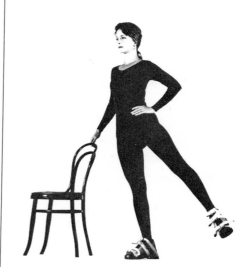

21 • Leg Lifts with Boots

This exercise firms and slims the hips.

Wearing 3-lb. boots, hold on to the back of a chair with your right hand and lift your left leg forward as high as you can.

Lower your leg to the floor. Then lift it out to the side.

Lower your leg again. Then lift it back behind you.

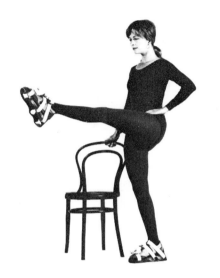

Return to your original position.

When doing this exercise, be sure to keep your legs straight and, for

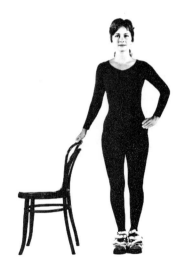

61

maximum results, use a kicking motion to raise your leg as high as possible.

Repeat 5 times with each leg. Gradually increase to 10.

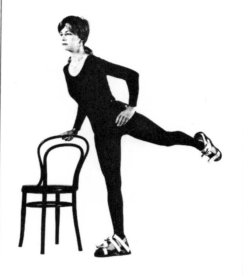

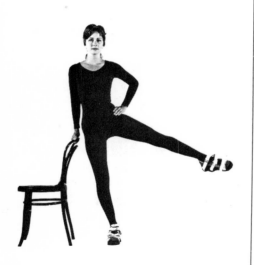

This ends the Beginner's Program. After four weeks, if you prefer to continue with these exercises, by all means do so. Only start the Intermediate series when you feel ready for heavier weights. On the other hand, you may wish to start the next series sooner, which is fine, if you work into it gradually, selecting only those exercises which you can perform without strain.

The Intermediate Program

By now you are well tuned in to all the muscles in your body. With each session you have felt them becoming firmer and stronger, and you have noticed that in your daily work and activities your energy level is higher, your body slimmer and more alive, and your mental outlook brighter.

In the Intermediate Program, the emphasis is on the lower body—the hips, buttocks, and thighs where many women have the most difficulty toning up and slimming down. If you feel that parts of your upper body need special strengthening and firming, then select exercises from the Beginner's Program that seem most beneficial to you and incorporate them here.

Intermediates use heavier weights and repeat the exercises a few more times than Beginners, so at this stage a new term, *sets,* is introduced. A set is the number of repetitions you must perform in each exercise. For example, *2 sets of 10* means to repeat the exercise 10 times, then STOP, breathe deeply for a moment, let the muscles rest briefly, and then continue on to the next set of 10 more repetitions. You'll find that these little breaks between sets will increase your efficiency and overall endurance.

After four weeks you will be ready to proceed to the Advanced Program. If you wish to stay on the Intermediate Program for a few more weeks, do so. Or if you find that this level is the one best suited to you, you can continue with the Intermediate Program indefinitely and still lose inches of unwanted fat. The critical factor is to continue exercising consistently.

Here is your exercise checklist for quick reference:

Warm-Ups
1. Run in place for one minute.
2. Dumbbell Swings: 1 5-lb. weight, repeat 10 to 15 times.
3. Dumbbell Bends: 2 10-lb. weights, do up to 2 sets of 12.

Upper Body
4. Barbell Bench Press: 10-lb. bar, do up to 2 sets of 12.
5. Bent Arm Lateral: 2 10-lb. weights, do up to 2 sets of 10.
6. Dumbbell Pullover: 1 10-lb. weight, do up to 3 sets of 12.

Waist and Stomach
7. Leg Raises: do up to 3 sets of 12.
8. Twisting Sit-Ups: do up to 2 sets of 15.
9. Half Squats: 10-lb. bar, do up to 3 sets of 10.

Hips, Thighs, and Legs

10. Leg Extension Back: 5-lb. boots, repeat 7 to 15 times each leg.
11. Leg Raises on Side: 5-lb. boots, repeat 7 to 15 times each leg.
12. Leg Lifts from Bench: 5-lb. boots, repeat 7 to 15 times each leg.
13. Leg Circles: 5-lb. boots, repeat 7 to 15 times each leg.
14. Leg Lifts with Boots: 5-lb. boots, repeat 10 times each leg.
15. Seated Leg Scissors: *no* boots, up to 2 sets of 15.
16. Adductor Presses with Ball: repeat 2 times.

1 • Run in place

Start with one minute and build up to two minutes.

2 • Dumbbell Swings *

This is the same exercise you performed in the Beginner's Program (p. 40).

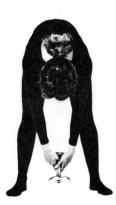

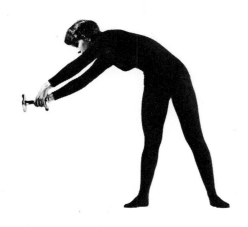

Be sure to make the circle wide. As you stretch, you will feel the tightness around your waist gradually disappear.

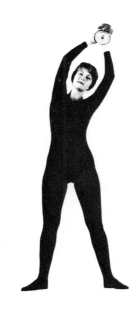

Regardless of how strong you are feeling, never use more than a 5-lb. weight for this exercise.

Repeat 10 times. Gradually increase to 15.

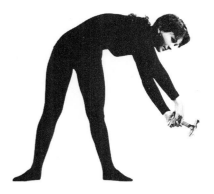

* If you have back problems, replace this exercise with the special back exercises on pages 109-112.

3 • *Dumbbell Bends*

This is the same exercise you performed in the Beginner's Program
(p. 42), but now you are ready to
use a 10-lb. weight in each hand.

Relax your neck and let the weight
stretch and firm your hip muscles.

Bending to the right and then to
the left, work up to 2 sets of 12.

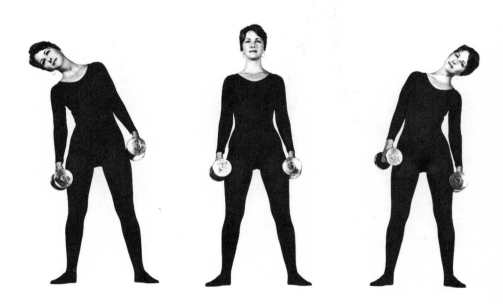

4 • Barbell Bench Press

This exercise relaxes tense shoulder muscles, strengthens pectoral muscles, and lifts the bustline. It also strengthens arm muscles.

It is similar to Exercise 4 in the Beginner's Program (p. 43), except that you will now use a 10-lb. bar.

Lie on your back on a bench, holding the bar up over your chest and keeping your arms straight.

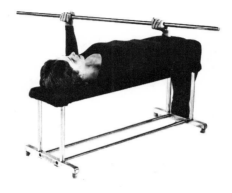

Inhale deeply and bring the bar down to your chest.

Exhale while raising your arms back to the starting position.

To firm and tone your arm muscles, hold the bar with a narrow grip (hands shoulder-width apart). To strengthen and firm chest muscles, move your hands further apart in a wider grip.

Work up to 2 sets of 12.

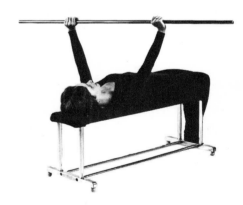

69

5 • Bent Arm Lateral

This is the same exercise you performed in the Beginner's Program (p. 44), but now you are ready to use a 10-lb. weight in each hand.

Remember to inhale deeply as you lower your arms to the sides and to exhale as you bring them back up.

Work up to 2 sets of 10.

70

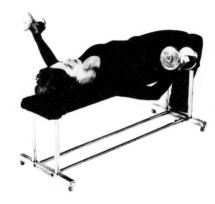

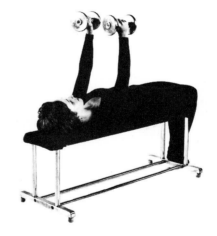

6 • Dumbbell Pullover

This exercise slims and firms the midriff and the backs of the arms and relaxes tense shoulder muscles.

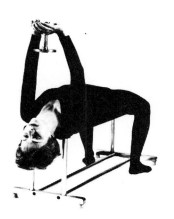

Lie on your back on a bench with your head hanging over the end of the bench.

Grasp a 10-lb. weight with both hands and hold your arms straight above your head.

Inhale slowly and deeply as you lower the weight back and over your head as far as possible without straining, keeping your arms straight.

Exhale completely as you bring your arms back up to the overhead starting position, again making sure that your arms remain straight.

Do this exercise as many times as you can without straining. Gradually work up to 3 sets of 12.

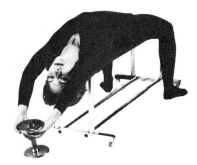

71

7 • Leg Raises *

This exercise strengthens abdominal muscles quickly and flattens the stomach.

Lie on your back on a bench with your legs hanging down from the bench at mid-thigh. Hold on to the bench with hands at hip level to keep your back pressed down against the bench.

Keeping your legs straight, raise them up and back over your head if you can.

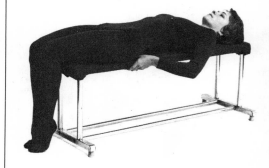

Now lower them *slowly* down to starting position.

You can also do this exercise on the floor. In that case keep your hands under your hips.

Work up to 3 sets of 12.

* If you have back problems, replace this exercise with the special back exercises on pages 109-112.

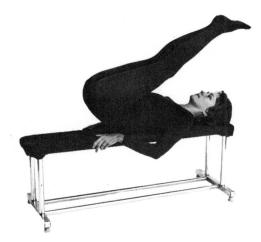

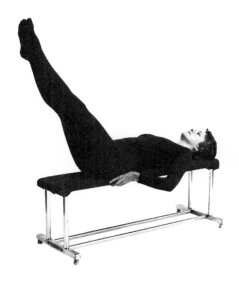

8 • Twisting Sit-Ups

This is the same exercise you performed in the Beginner's Program (p. 51), but now you are strong enough to do more of them. Each time you perform this exercise, strive to increase the number of sit-ups beyond 10.

Your goal should be 2 sets of 15.

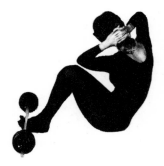

9 • *Half Squats*

This exercise firms and strengthens most of the muscles in the body and is especially helpful for slimming the abdominal area. It also benefits posture and is excellent for improving balance.

Place a 10-lb. bar across shoulders behind your head. Stand with your feet shoulder-width apart.

Turn your feet out far enough so that when you bend your knees, you cannot see your big toe. Correct position is important for the protection of the knee joint.

With back held straight, bend your knees and squat halfway down, no further.

Now straighten up to starting position.

Work up to 3 sets of 10.

Try to increase the weight gradually to 20 lb.

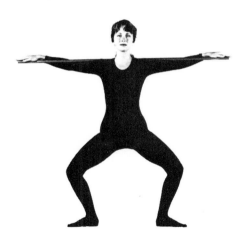

10 • Leg Extension Back *

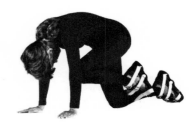

This is the same exercise you per-formed in the Beginner's Program (p. 57), but now you are ready to use 5-lb. boots.

Repeat 7 times with each leg. Gradually increase to 15.

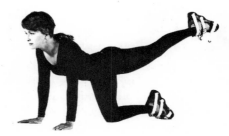

* If you have back problems, replace this exer-cise with the special back exercises on pages 109-112.

76

11 • *Leg Raises on Side*

This is the same exercise you performed in the Beginner's Program (p. 58), but now you are ready to use 5-lb. boots.

To enhance your stamina and make the exercise easier, inhale deeply each time you raise your leg and exhale as you lower it.

Repeat 7 times with each leg. Gradually increase to 15.

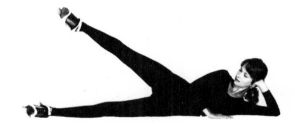

77

12 • Leg Lifts from Bench

This is the same exercise you performed in the Beginner's Program (p. 59), but now you are ready to use 5-lb. boots.

Repeat 7 times with each leg. Gradually increase to 15.

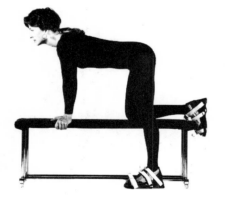

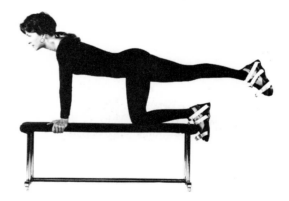

13 • Leg Circles

This is the same exercise you performed in the Beginner's Program (p. 60), but now you are ready to use 5-lb. boots.

As you strive to widen the circles that you make with your leg, the slimming effectiveness of this exercise increases impressively.

Repeat 7 times with each leg. Gradually increase to 15.

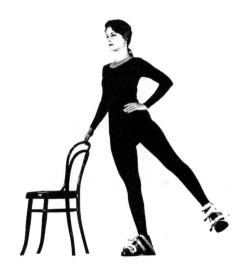

79

14 • Leg Lifts with Boots

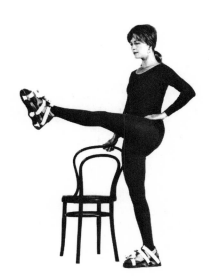

This is the same exercise you performed in the Beginner's Program (p. 61), but now you are ready to use 5-lb. boots.

Kick and lift as high as you can and feel the energy pulse through your body.

Repeat 10 times with each leg.

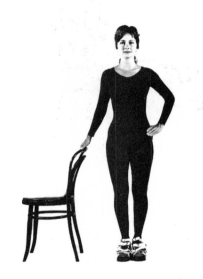 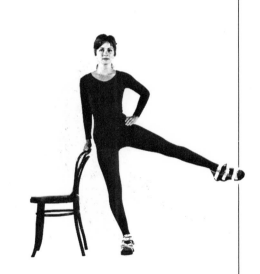 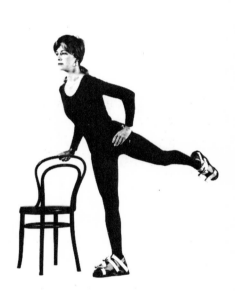

81

15 • Seated Leg Scissors

This exercise strengthens all muscles in the lower body. It is especially good for slimming the inner thighs and for flattening the stomach.

Take the boots off and sit down on a bench or chair.

Grip the bench firmly behind your back.

Keeping your legs straight, raise them as high as you can without leaning back too far.

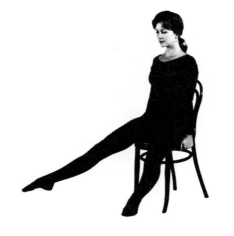

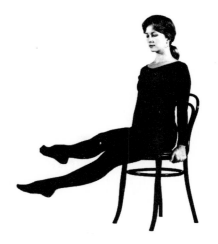

Spread your legs far apart; then crisscross them scissors fashion.

Work up to 2 sets of 15.

16 • Adductor Presses with Ball

This exercise strengthens the knees and ankles, and firms thighs and calves.

Sit on a bench or chair and place a big rubber ball between your thighs. (Any large round object will do—even foam rubber pillows—as long as you squeeze hard.)

Holding on to the bench behind your back, straighten your legs out in front of you. Do not lean back too far.

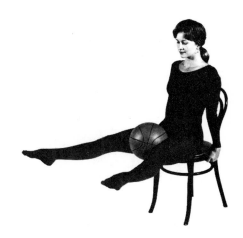

Squeeze the ball with your thighs continuously for 6 seconds.

Now place the ball between your knees and squeeze it there for 6 seconds.

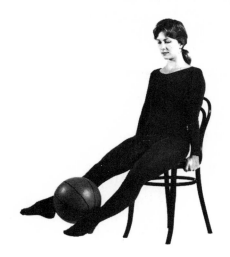

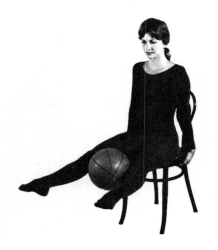

Now place the ball between your ankles and squeeze for 6 seconds.

Repeat this sequence once more.

The Advanced Program

At this stage you have accomplished a great many goals. You are now in the habit of exercising with weights on a regular basis; you have become aware of the awesome way every muscle in your body has reacted to tone up your body and increase your energy; you have lost inches in places you never thought you could lose them before; and your strength has increased dramatically. These changes show. You are relaxed and mentally alert, and you move more gracefully and perform daily tasks much more easily and quickly than ever before.

Now you are ready to progress to heavier weights in a more challenging program of exercise that will increase all these benefits. And you will find that even after you have lost all the inches you needed to lose or toned up your body to its peak capacity, you'll want to continue—in fact you'll miss it if you don't exercise. Many women find they even want to increase weight sizes beyond the Advanced stage. In this, as in all other stages of development, the rule is to *go slowly*. Build yourself up to extra weights gradually, and if you feel any strain or pain at all, then STOP and use lighter weights until your body is fully prepared to handle the heavier weights.

Happily, then, the Advanced Program never ends, and neither do its benefits. After four weeks you'll be amazed to remember the old fatigued and unshapely you who began this program as a Beginner, and you'll continue exercising with weights every other day for the rest of your life.

Here is your exercise checklist for quick reference:

Warm-Ups
1. Run in place for 2 minutes.
2. Dumbbell Swings: 1 5-lb. weight, do 2 sets of 10.
3. Dumbbell Bends: 2 16-lb. weights, do up to 2 sets of 15.

Upper Body
4. Barbell Bench Press: 20-lb. bar, do up to 2 sets of 12.
5. Arm Raises: 2 3-lb. weights, do up to 2 sets of 10.
6. Dips from Bench: do up to 2 sets of 10.
7. Barbell Curls: 16-lb. bar, do up to 3 sets of 10.

Waist and Stomach
8. Bar Twist Seated: 20-lb. bar, do up to 2 sets of 20.
9. Half Squats: 20-lb. bar, do up to 2 sets of 10.
10. Twisting Sit-Ups: do up to 20 times.

Hips, Thighs, and Legs

11. Thigh Turns: repeat 10 times.
12. Leg Extension Back: 5-lb. boots, repeat 10 to 20 times.
13. Leg Raises on Side: 5-lb. boots, repeat 10 to 20 times each leg.
14. Leg Lifts from Bench: 5-lb. boots, repeat 10 to 20 times each leg.
15. Leg Circles: 5-lb. boots, repeat 10 to 20 times each leg.
16. Leg Lifts with Boots: 5-lb. boots, repeat 10 to 15 times each leg.
17. Leg Circles on Stomach: 5-lb. boots, repeat 10 to 15 times each leg.
18. Leg Circles on Back: 5-lb. boots, repeat 10 to 15 times each leg.
19. Leg Crossovers: 5-lb. boots, repeat 10 to 15 times each leg.
20. Seated Leg Scissors: 5-lb. boots, repeat up to 10 times.
21. Side Lunges with Barbell: 20-lb. bar, do 2 sets of 10.
22. Leg Thrusts: *no* boots, do up to 2 sets of 10.

1 • Run in place

Start with 2 minutes and work up to as many minutes as you have time and endurance for.

2 • Dumbbell Swings *

As in the Intermediate Program (p. 66), make wide circles with your arms while holding a 5-lb. weight with both hands.

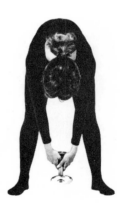

Stretch and stretch to make that circle as wide as you can without straining.

Do 2 sets of 10.

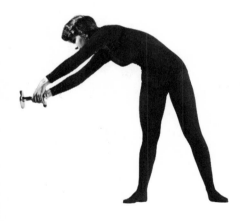

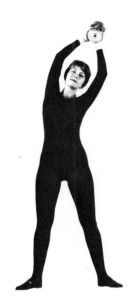

* As before, if you still have back problems, replace this exercise with the special back exercises on pages 109-112.

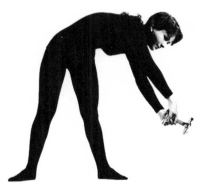

3 • Dumbbell Bends

This is the same exercise you performed in the Intermediate Program (p. 68), but now you are ready to use 16-lb. weights as you bend from side to side.

Notice tension disappear as waist and hip muscles stretch.

Work up to 2 sets of 15.

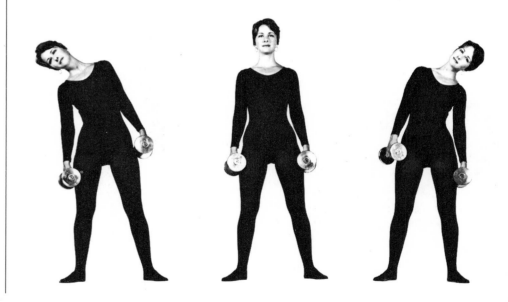

4 • Barbell Bench Press

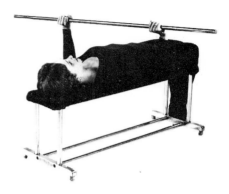

This exercise relaxes tense shoulders, firms chest and arm muscles, and lifts the bustline.

This is the same exercise you performed in the Intermediate Program (p. 69), but now you are ready to use a 20-lb. bar.

Breathe deeply—feel your chest expand and your chest muscles tighten.

Work up to 2 sets of 12.

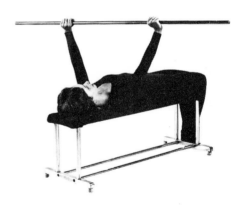

91

5 • Arm Raises

This exercise slims arms and strengthens shoulders.

Hold a 3-lb. weight in each hand and stand with your feet wide apart for good balance.

Bend forward at the waist until your back is parallel to the floor.

Start with your arms hanging down in front of you and the palms of your hands facing each other.

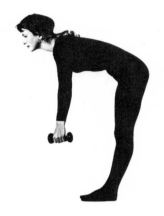

Inhale as you raise your arms out to the sides and up until they are level with your shoulders—*no higher.*

Exhale as you slowly lower your arms to starting position.

Work up to 2 sets of 10.

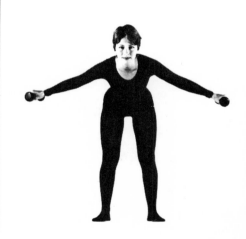

6 • Dips from Bench

This exercise slims and firms the back of the upper arms.

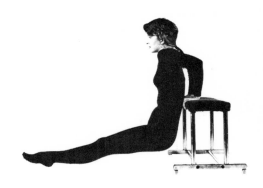

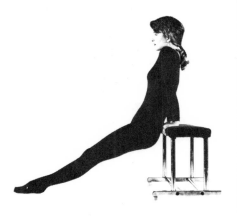

This is similar to the exercise you performed in the Beginner's Program (p. 48). As before, sit on the edge of the bench and lower your body almost to the floor, but this time keep your legs straight.

Work up to 2 sets of 10.

7 • Barbell Curls

This exercise strengthens arm muscles tremendously.

Stand holding a 16-lb. barbell with hands about shoulder-width apart. The palms of your hands should face away from your body.

Inhale and raise the bar up toward your shoulders.

Now exhale as you lower the bar to starting position.

94

Be sure to keep your back straight while you do this exercise. Your forearms should do the work, *not* your back.

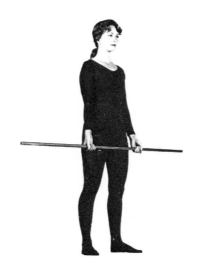

Watch your arms, and you will see the muscles firm with each lift.

Work up to 3 sets of 10.

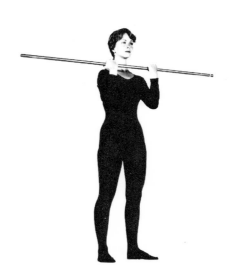

8 • Bar Twist Seated

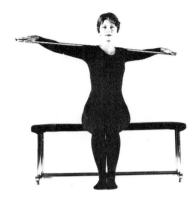

This is the same exercise you performed in the Beginner's Program (p. 50), but now you are ready to use a 20-lb. barbell.

Sit on a bench with the bar across your shoulders, and twist from side to side at the waist.

Twist rhythmically and at a moderate speed—you will feel your upper waist firming and slimming with each twist.

Work up to 2 sets of 20.

95

9 • Half Squats

This exercise firms and strengthens most of the muscles in the body and is especially helpful for slimming the abdominal area. It also benefits posture and improves balance.

It is the same exercise that you performed in the Intermediate Program (p. 75), but now you are ready to use a 20-lb. bar.

Be sure to keep your back straight and do not squat lower than halfway down.

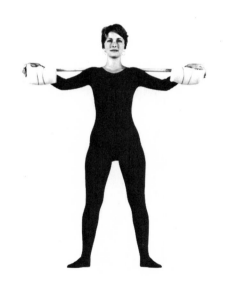

You'll begin to feel your posture and balance improve dramatically after only a few weeks of this exercise.

Work up to 2 sets of 10.

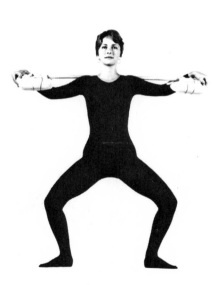

10 • Twisting Sit-Ups

This exercise slims the waist and strengthens the stomach muscles.

This is the same exercise you performed in the Intermediate Program (p. 74), but now you are ready to elevate your feet on a low chair. You can also use a slant board, if you have one.

Do as many as you can, gradually building up to 20 repetitions.

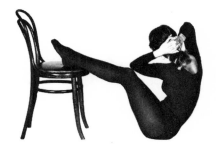

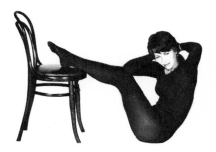

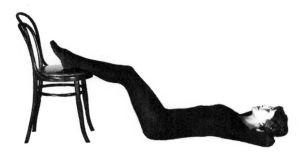

11 • Thigh Turns

This exercise firms and slims the inner thighs. It also strengthens the lower abdominal muscles.

Sit on the floor with your legs stretched out in front of you and apart.

Put your arms behind you and lean back on your elbows.

Raise your legs about a foot off the floor and twist your thighs in toward each other; then twist them out.

The motion should come from the lower hip area—try not to move the pelvis.

Repeat 10 times.

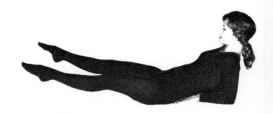

12–16 • Boot Exercises

Wearing 5-lb. boots, do all of the boot exercises from the Intermediate Program (exercises 10–14), beginning on p. 76. Then add the following 3 new boot exercises.

17 • Leg Circles on Stomach

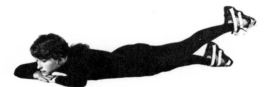

This exercise firms thighs and buttocks.

Wearing 5-lb. boots, lie face down on the floor with your hands under your chin.

Lift your right leg a few inches off the floor and make small circles with your foot as close to the floor as possible.

Repeat 10 times with each leg. Gradually increase to 15.

18 • Leg Circles on Back

This exercise strengthens the stomach muscles and firms the thighs.

With 5-lb. boots on, lie on your back and make small circles with your right leg a few inches off the floor.

Repeat 10 times with each leg. Gradually increase to 15.

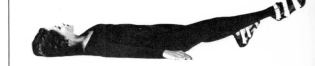

19 • Leg Crossovers

This exercise firms the inner thighs and the hips.

Wearing the 5-lb. boots and lying on your back, raise your legs straight up toward the ceiling.

Keeping your legs straight, crisscross them. Then extend them as far apart as you can.

Return to starting position with your legs pointing straight up.

For maximum slimming results, do this exercise slowly.

Repeat 10 times. Gradually increase to 15.

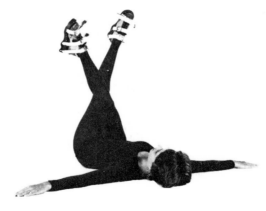
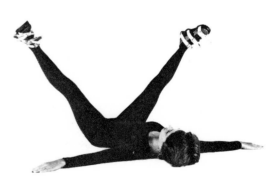

20 • Seated Leg Scissors

This is the same exercise you performed in the Intermediate Program (p. 82), but now you are ready to do it wearing 5-lb. boots.

This exercise is rather strenuous, so start out slowly and work up to 10 repetitions.

You'll feel it firming and strengthening your inner thighs and abdominal muscles every time you cross your legs.

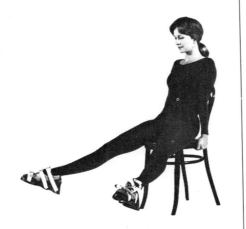

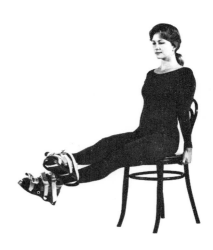

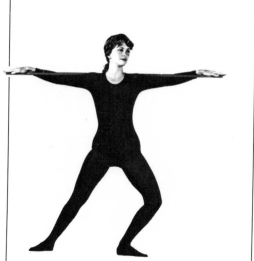

21 • Side Lunges with Barbell

This exercise slims and firms thighs. It is also excellent for toning and smoothing those "dimpled" or "puckered" areas of fatty tissue that plague many women.

Standing with your feet close together, hold a 20-lb. bar across your shoulders behind your head.

Turn your right foot out and take a big step to the side, bending your knee as you put your foot down.

Bring your right foot back to starting position and repeat with the left leg.

Do 2 sets of 10.

22 • Leg Thrusts

This exercise increases overall endurance and strengthens arms and legs.

On your hands and knees on the floor, rest your weight on your arms, keeping them straight throughout the exercise.

Stretch one leg out behind you; bend the other leg and bring it close to your chest.

With a thrust or jump, reverse the position of your legs.

Work up to 2 sets of 10.

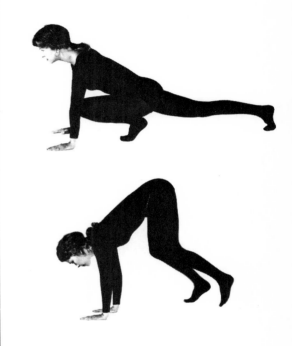

Appendix of Special Exercises

This group of simple exercises focuses on those parts of the body that seem particularly vulnerable to aches and pain—the back, stomach, and knees. They are not intended as a cure for severe problems, and if you are under a physician's care, you definitely should see her or him before doing them.

These exercises are excellent for strengthening the back muscles and for alleviating strain, aches, and tension. Try to do them for a few minutes every day.

SPECIAL BACK EXERCISES

1. Lie on your back on the floor.

Keeping your right leg flat on the floor, draw your left leg up toward your chest.

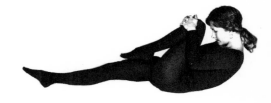

Grasp your left knee with your hands and pull it against your chest. Hold this position for 5 seconds.

Alternate legs and repeat 10 or more times.

2. Lie on your back on the floor.

Put your hands around your knees and draw your knees up to your chest.

Spread your knees as far apart as possible.

Press your back to the floor, raise your head, and press your chin toward your chest.

Hold for 5 seconds.

Relax and repeat.

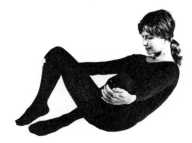

3. Get down on your hands and knees.

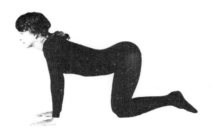

Take a deep breath, hold your stomach in, and arch your back like a Halloween cat.

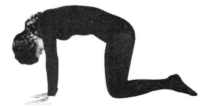

4. Hang from a chinning bar for 5 seconds. (If you have a disc problem, *do not* do this exercise without permission from your physician.)

Your feet should clear the floor, but do not jump to get on and off the bar. Instead, use a stool for getting on and off.

This exercise is very helpful for strengthening weak backs. It also relaxes every muscle in the body.

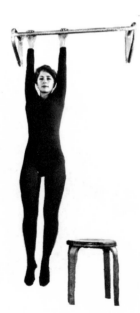

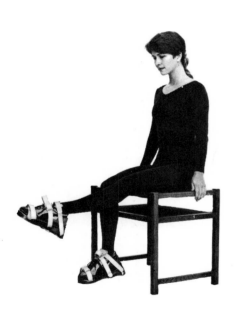

SPECIAL KNEE EXERCISE

5. Wearing 3-lb. boots, sit on the edge of a table. Make sure that the backs of your knees are right at the table's edge.

Start with your legs hanging down. Lift your left leg slowly until it is parallel to the table.

Then lower it and lift your right leg up.

Repeat several times.

After you have completed the Beginner's Program, you may do this exercise with 5-lb. boots.

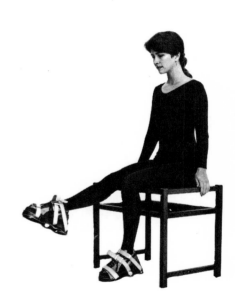

113

SPECIAL STOMACH EXERCISES

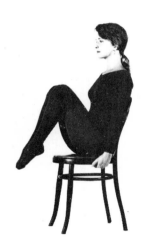

6. Sit on the edge of a chair. Draw your knees up to your chest and hold onto the seat of the chair with your hands.

Now extend your legs in front of you. Do not let them drop to the floor. Hold them there for five seconds.

Return to the starting position with feet on the floor.

Repeat 8 times.

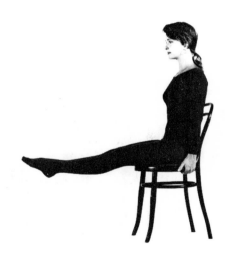

114

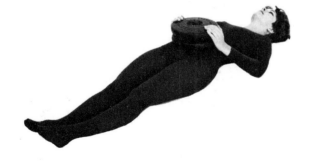

7. Lie on your back on the floor.

Place a 20-lb. weight (a few heavy books will do) on your stomach.

Holding the weight in place with your hands, take a deep breath and push the weight up with your stomach muscles.

Exhale and relax the stomach muscles.

Repeat several times.

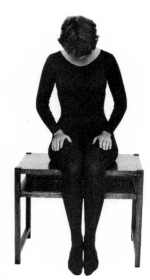

SPECIAL EXERCISES FOR TENSION

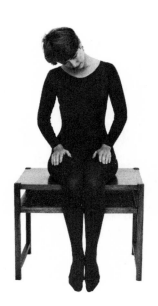

8. Sit down. Roll your head in a clockwise circle from left to right. Repeat 10 times.

Reverse direction, and repeat 10 more times.

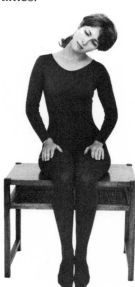

9. Stand with your arms hanging down.

Starting from the back and moving forward, make large circles with your shoulders.

Repeat 10 times.

Then reverse directions and circle from front to back.

Repeat 10 times.

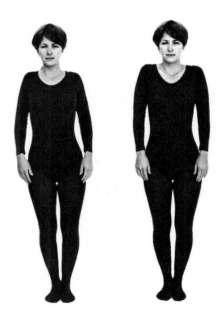

Acknowledgments

In many ways this book is a combined effort. It could not have been written without the help of Skip Arroyo, who designed, tested, and improved upon her weight-exercise program for many years. I am also grateful for the constant patience and cooperation of our model, Jody Taylor, who was able to hold strenuous positions, shot after shot, with amazing composure and grace. Less visible behind-the-scenes help came from photographer Ted Streshinsky, who offered valuable technical advice, and from my editor, Pat Holt, who was extremely supportive from beginning to end.

119